DIY Bath Bombs:

Step-By-Step Beginner's Guide To Making Bath Bombs

With 30 Amazing All-Natural Bath Bomb Recipes

Table of content:

Introduction - You're ready to get started...

You've downloaded the book, and now you're ready to get started with a new hobby that will have you spoiling yourself and your friends and family. I can walk you through the process every step of the way. I have formatted this book to:

• Give you a list of tools you will need to make them

• Give you a list of ingredients you will need and how to get them

• Explain how to use dyes and powders to color your bath bombs

• List the differences between using fragrances and essential oils

• List the essential oils you will need for the bath bombs.

• List recipes you can try with the essential oils in the bath bombs.

So, if you're ready, swipe the page and let's get to it!

Chapter 1 - Intro to Bath Bombs

Bath bombs are a great way to relax at the end of the day.

The way it fizzes relaxes the mind and a good soak in the tub does wonders for the body, but what do you need to make them? Why does it fizz? We will look into that.

Tools of the trade

Just like any other hobby, you will need the proper tools to make bath bombs. Luckily, you probably have most of them in your kitchen.

• Kitchen scale

• Glass/metal mixing bowls

• Silicone or plastic mixing spoons

• Sifter-the powders you use will have to be sifted to mix properly

• Spray bottle

• Molds- These can be silicone, glass, plastic or metal

• Storage containers-to store your bath bombs

• Labels-to keep your bath bombs organized

Ingredients

Now, for what you will need to purchase to get started.

● Citric Acid

● Baking Soda

● Fragrance oils or essential oils

● Witch Hazel

● Mica Dye powders (optional)

Fragrance oils v Essential oils

Fragrance oils are an inexpensive way to add light and pleasing aromas to your bath bombs. They are artificially manufactured more often than not, which can lead to some allergic reactions in sensitive skins and people with allergies to artificial additives.

Essential oils are derived from plants and can have therapeutic effects when you use them in bath bombs and other preparations. This does mean you will be spending a little more in order to make the bath bomb, but you will have all-natural, high-quality and therapeutic aromas in them.

The choice is ultimately up to you.

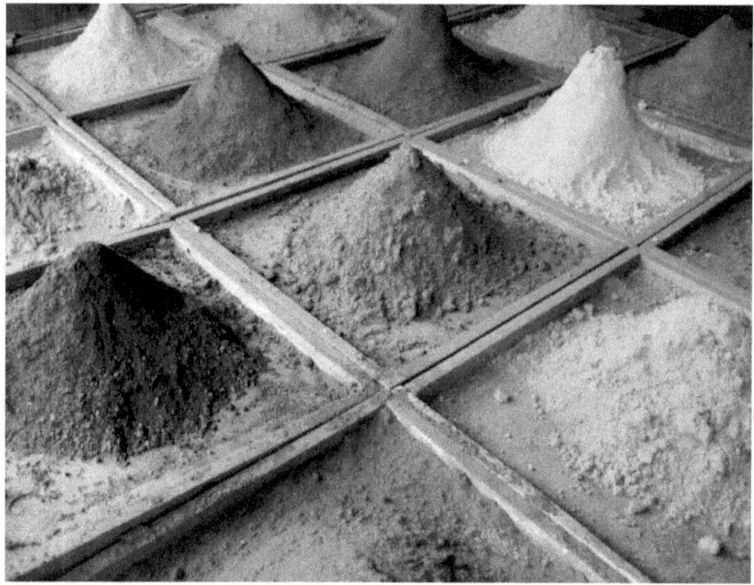

Mica is a natural mineral which comes in a wide variety of colors as well as having had colorants added to them. A reputable vendor will let you know if the mica is naturally that color or if it has had color added to it. When you add the mica to the powders, it will retain its color, but it may be lighter or darker depending on how much you add to the mixture. Baking soda and Citric Acid are both white, so they will dilute even the strongest and brightest of color dyes.

Why does it fizz?

You have probably wondered why, when you put the bath bomb in water, it fizzes. When you combine baking soda and citric acid, they have a chemical reaction with the water to produce the bubbles and the fizz you see when you put the bath bomb in the tub. There is nothing to worry about. It's perfect safe.

Here is the basic recipe for the **bath bombs**:

Your mold-This can be a muffin pan
16 oz Citric Acid
32 oz Baking Soda
.75 oz Fragrance oil or essential oil blend (4 1/2 tsp)
Witch Hazel

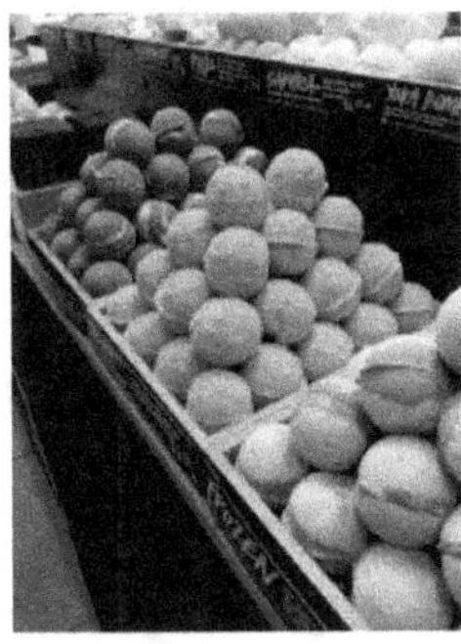

Mica dye

1.   Combine the citric acid fragrance and baking soda in the mixing bowl

2. Sift it to remove any lumps

3. Add the dye and mix until the desired color is reached

4. Spray the witch hazel until the mix is staying together when you squeeze it. It can crack if it is not moist enough. This will take practice.

5. Once it is staying together, place it in the mold. You will have to pack it tightly or it will crack.

6. It should not take more than 30 seconds for it to set in the mold.

Chapter 2 - Essential Oils

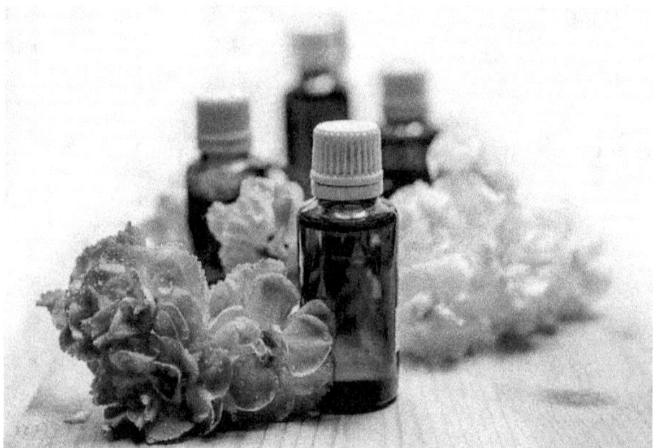

Essential oils are the distilled essence of the plant. There are over ninety (90) different essential oils and many more are being discovered, but we will touch on the ones that are more affordable in this book. Essential oils are the backbone of Aromatherapy. The perfect blend of essential oils can relax the nerves, soothe muscles, and tone skin. You can even blend the essential oils together to make perfumes and essences that can take you other places.

There are some things to take as a caution when dealing with essential oils.

1. Never use them undiluted. There are some companies out there who say it is perfectly fine to use essential oils undiluted. This is simply not true. Undiluted essentials oils can cause contact dermatitis. Even Lavender, which has been used sparingly undiluted can cause this condition when used to much and too often.

2. Use gloves when mixing essential oils.

3. Keep essential oils out of the reach of children. Essential oils can be toxic in large doses and should not be anywhere near small children.

4. Store essential oils in a cool, dry location. Due to the nature of essential oils, if they are exposed to heat, they can evaporate in the bottle, leaving you with an empty essential oil bottle and a lot of disappointment.

5. Blend the essential oils before you add them to the dry ingredients. You want the synergy of the essentials to be there before you add them to the baking soda citric acid.

6. Do a patch test. Dilute three drops of an essential oil in one teaspoon of vegetable oil and work it into a small patch of skin. If you do not have a reaction to it within 24 hours, it is safe for you to use.

You will notice that I include the Latin name for the essential oils that are most used for each type of bath bomb. This is because one plant name can reference many different plants and including the Latin name makes sure you can get the exact essential oil for your needs. Now, on to the recipes.

Chapter 3 - Relaxing Bath Bombs

Stress, we all deal with it on a daily basis. Whether it's meeting deadlines, managing money, balancing work with personal life or having to deal with all of it at once, stress is an ever-present facet of our lives. There are things you can do to help tame it and manage it.

Spoil Yourself

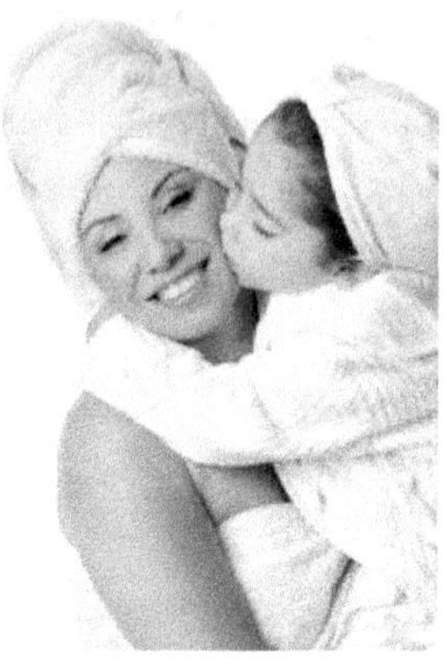

Once a day for about 30 minutes, do something you want to do. Read a book; meditate; or take a long, relaxing bath. You can even listen to soothing music while you soak your muscles in hot bath. Just make sure you there are no distractions. Don't feel the least bit guilty either. Everyone deserves to spoil themselves. It's part of taking care of you.

Exercise

This can be as simple as taking a walk or going to gym and taking a kickboxing class. Exercise has been proven to reduce and relieve stress. Find an exercise you like, and you will more apt to stick with it.

Unplug

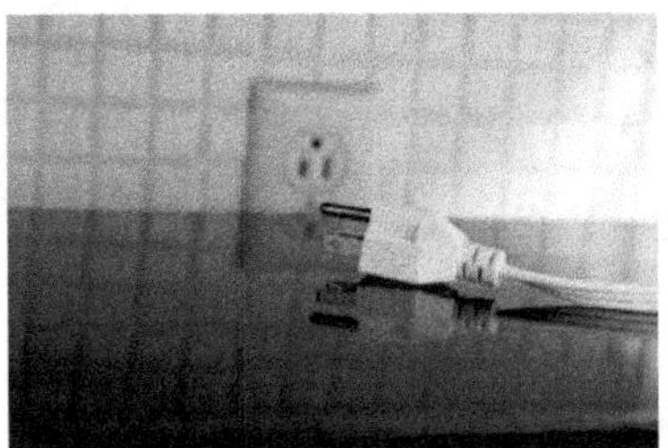

We live in a world where information is constantly at our fingertips. Texts, looking up information, emails, it's all stimulus for the brain, and taking a break from all of it can relax your brain and relieve stress. So, turn off the laptop/desktop, turn off the smartphone, and avoid any electronics for about 15 minutes. Give your mind a rest.

Listen to soothing music/ambient sounds

Otherwise known as white noise, listening to ambient sounds can relax the mind and in turn, the body as well. Soothing music, like sooth jazz, can relieve stress, too.

Anxiety

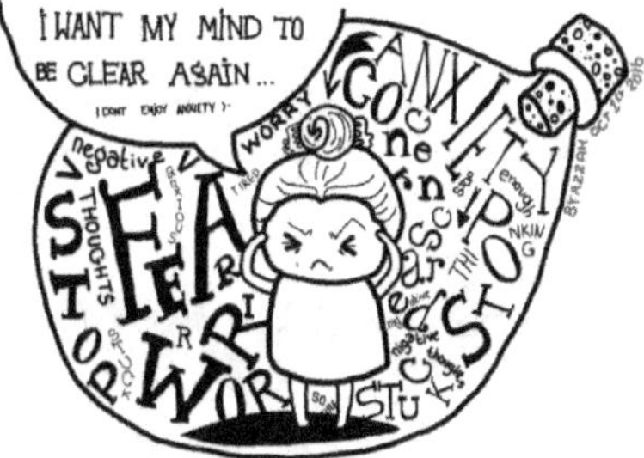

That tightness in the chest, the panic that sets in, the gasping for air, it feels like your having a heart attack, but it's anxiety, intense anxiety, and it can be crippling. You can learn to manage your anxiety by going to your doctor, visiting a psychologist and even trying the following:

Take breaks

When things start to get to be too much, step away from it and take a break. This goes for being at work, too. Take those 15 minute breaks and lunches.

Get plenty of sleep

On average 6-8 hours of sleep is ideal and can help with anxiety.

Eat a balanced diet

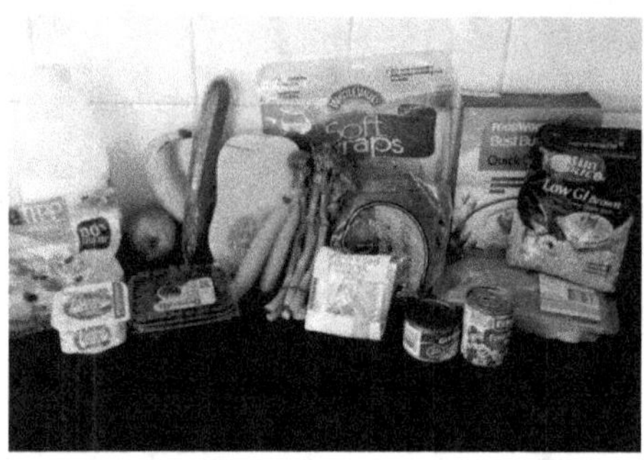

Whole foods and a balanced diet can help reduce the instances of anxiety or anxiety attacks.

Cut down or cut out caffeine

Any drink that has caffeine can possibly trigger an anxiety attack.

Learn your triggers

Learning and writing down your triggers will help you void them in the future. By avoiding the triggers, you can reduce the incidents of anxiety attacks.

Find the Funny

In every situation there is a grain of humor in it. Laughter can diffuse an anxiety-ridden situation. Try to find the "funny" in the situation.

Exercise

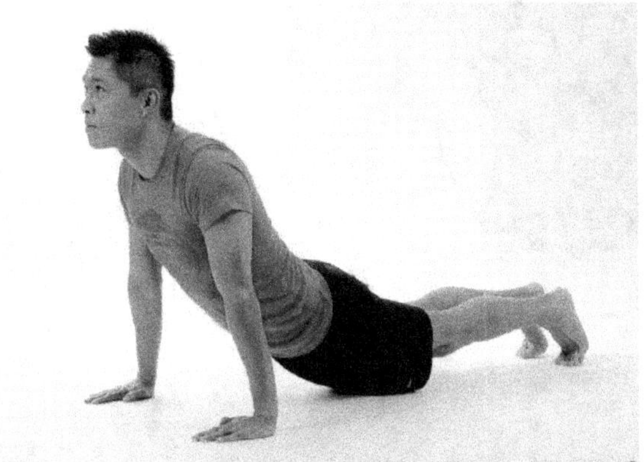

This can work wonders for anxiety. It can tire you out and release any suppressed anxiety. Find an exercise or exercise routine you like and can stick with.

Talk to someone

We all need a shoulder to cry on and vent to when something tweaks our nerve. If you have someone in your circles you can talk to when you're feeling an anxiety attack coming on, then talk to them and it will help you calm down.

BERGAMOT (CITRUS BERGAMIA)

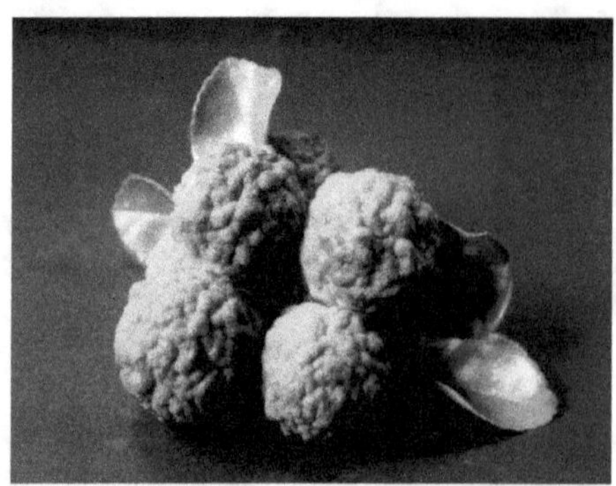

This citrus aroma can help relieve the feelings of anxiety and calm you from a stressful day. It can uplift the spirit and also help with depression.

CHAMOMILE, ROMAN (CHAMAEMELUM NOBILE)

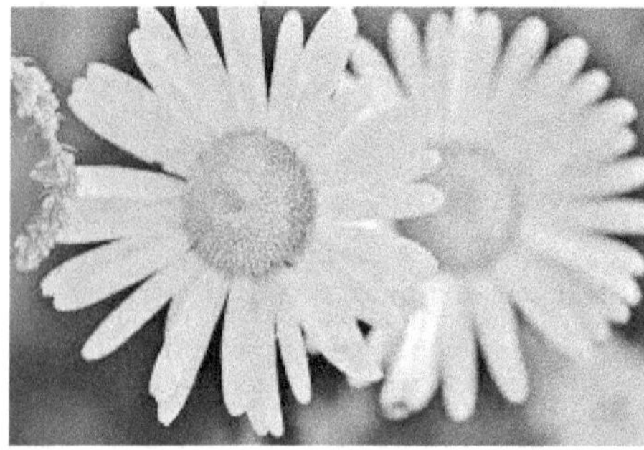

Just smelling the flowers of the herb can reduce tension. This is why chamomile is widely used in aromatherapy for stress and anxiety. It can also help you sleep if your having problems doing so.

FRANKINCENSE (BOSWELLIA CARTERI)

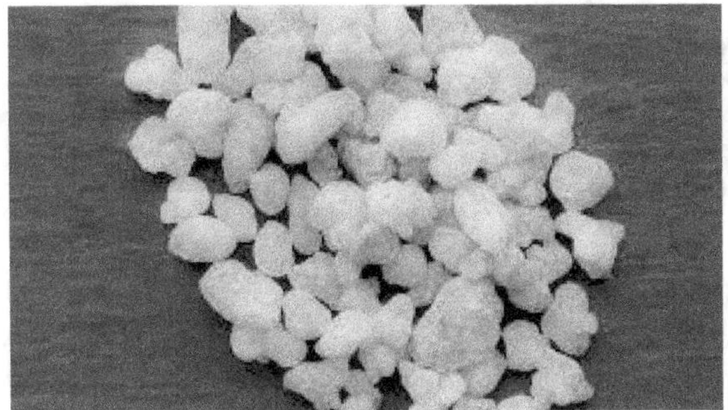

This essential oil comes from the resin many religions use for incense. It can soothe frayed nerves, calm the spirit and help you when you want to meditate. It is used for relieving stress and anxiety.

LAVENDER (LAVANDULA ANGUSTIFOLIA)

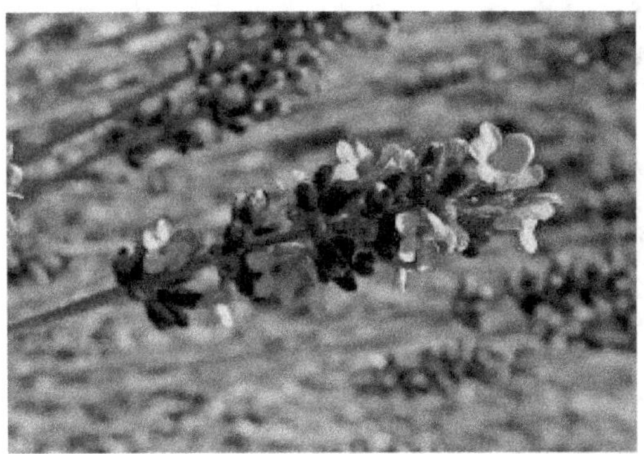

This is one of the first essential oils to be discovered. Just a whiff from the bottle can help to relieve stress and when you put it in an aromatherapy blend, it helps with anxiety, nervous tension and sleeping problems.

MARJORAM (ORIGANUM MARJORANA)

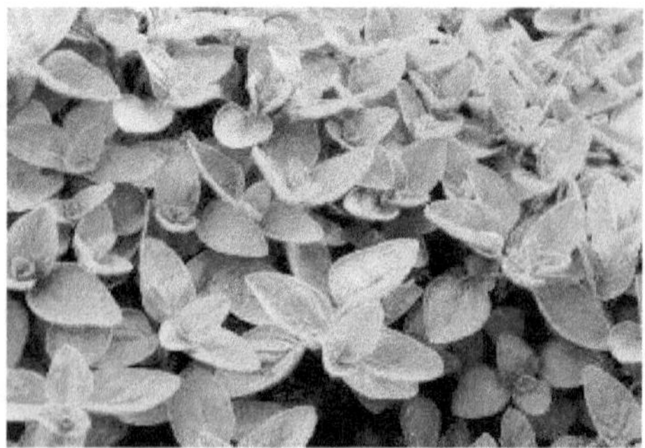

Most people would recognize this as an herb used in Italian dishes and to add a little pep to meat rubs. As an essential oil, it can help the body bounce back from stress-related conditions and help with nervous tension.

ROSE, DAMASK (ROSA X DAMASCENA)

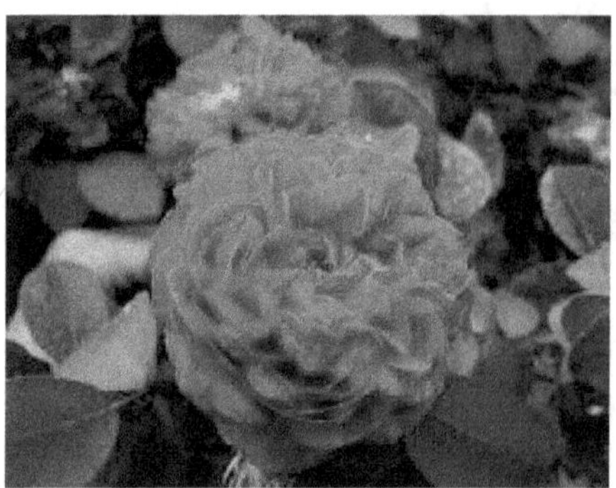

This is one of the more expensive essential oils as it takes a ton of rose petals to make one ounce of the oil. It works wonders for stress-related problems, nervous tension, and sleep disorders. It is also recommended to help with depression.

ROSEWOOD (ANIBA ROSAEODORA)

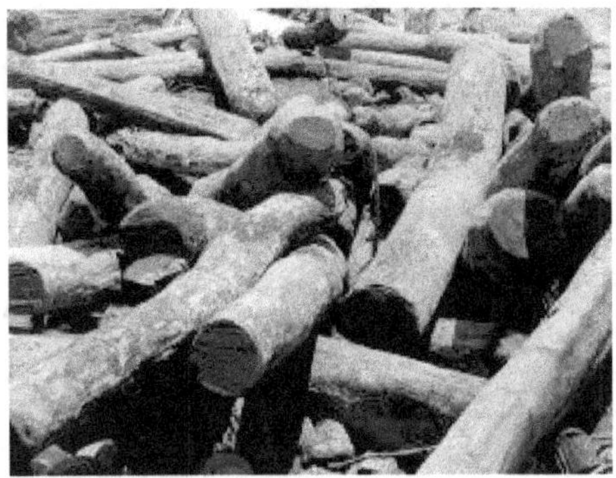

If you suffer from a lot of nervous tension and find yourself uncomfortable in many situations, try keeping a cotton ball with three drops of this essential oil on you. Take a whiff. This essential oil is great for relieving a case of the nerves and for helping with problems related to stress.

VETIVER (VETIVERIA ZIZANIODES)

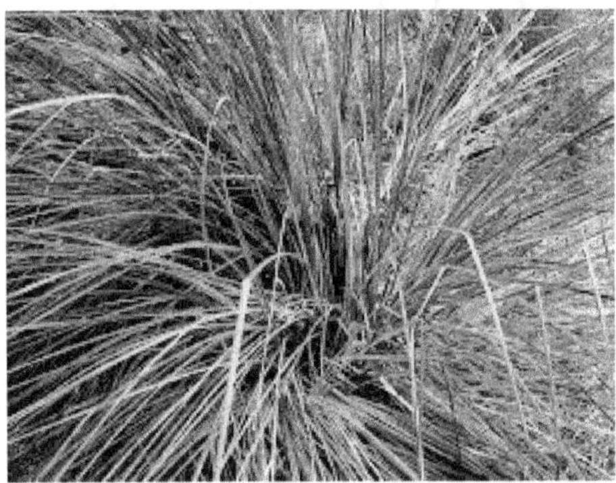

If you are having troubles sleeping due to stress or anxiety, this essential oil will be right up your alley.

YLANG YLANG (CANANGA ODORATA VAR. GENUINA)

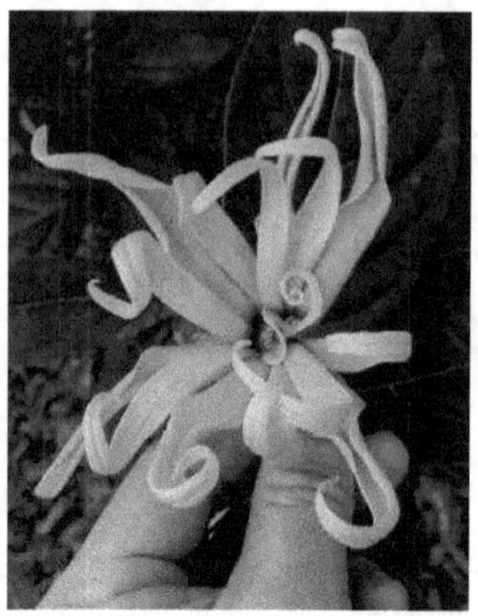

This is another pricey essential oil, but it's worth its price. It comes highly recommended in cases of nervous tension and disorders that come about due to stress. It's also wonderful for depression and insomnia.

Anxiety Formula I

2 tsp of Lavender essential oil
1 1/2 tsp of Chamomile essential oil
1/2 tsp of Vetiver essential oil
1/2 tsp of Frankincense essential oil

Anxiety formula II

.25 oz of Vanilla fragrance
.25 oz of Lavender Fragrance
.25 oz of Orange Fragrance

Anxiety formula III

.25 oz of Bergamot essential oil
.25 oz of Lavender essential oil
.25 oz of Ylang Ylang essential oil

Stress formula I

.25 oz of Rosewood essential oil
.15 oz of Marjoram essential oil
.35 oz of Bergamot essential oil

Stress formula II

.15 oz of Frankincense essential oil
.10 oz of Marjoram essential oil
.25 oz of Ylang Ylang essential oil
.25 oz of Rose, Damask essential oil

Stress formula III

.25 oz of Bergamot essential oil
.25 oz of Ylang Ylang essential oil
.25 oz of Chamomile essential oil

We all need to relax when we have finished out work for the day. The problem is finding the time to relax and just wind down from a long day. Here is a list of essential oils that can help with that.

GERANIUM (PELARGONIUM GRAVEOLENS)

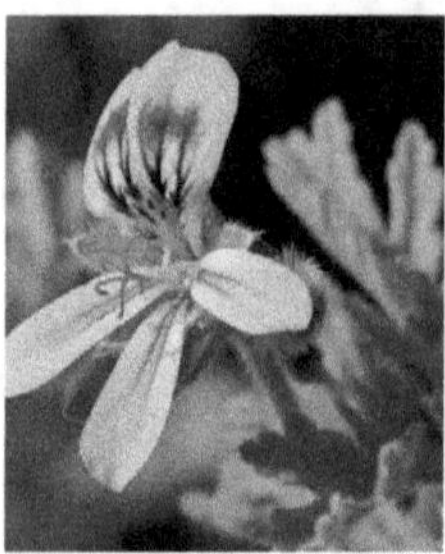

This essential oil is great for the end of the day when you need to de-stress and relax your mind. It's also good for nervous tension.

LEMON (CITRUS LIMON)

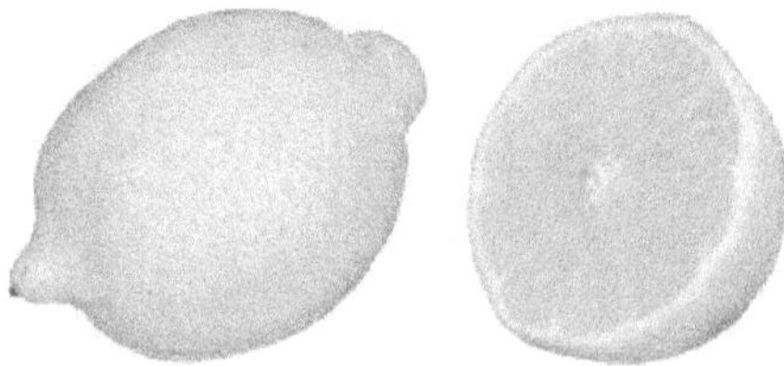

Just the smell of this essential oil can help to drain the stress of the day and help you wind down.

JASMINE (JASMINUM OFFICINALE)

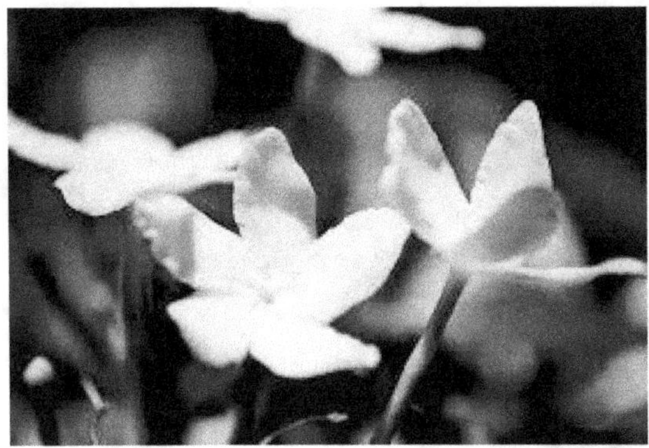

One of the more expensive essential oils, Jasmine works wonders for depression, exhaustion due to nerves and other stress-related conditions.

MANDARIN (CITRUS RETICULATA)

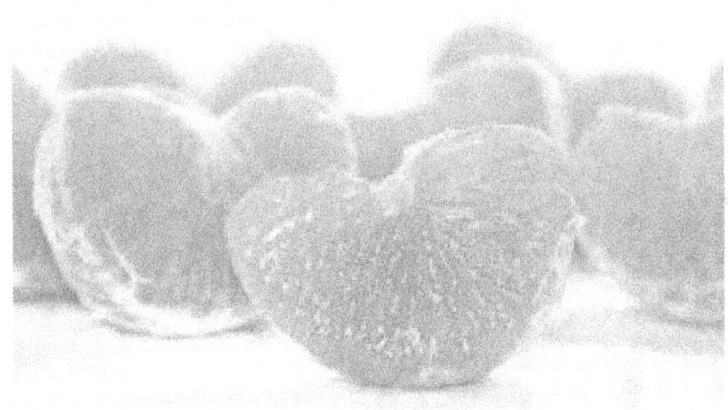

This citrus essential oil has an aroma that melts tension, relaxes the mind and get your body and mind ready for sleep.

PALMAROSA (CYMBOPOGON MARTINII)

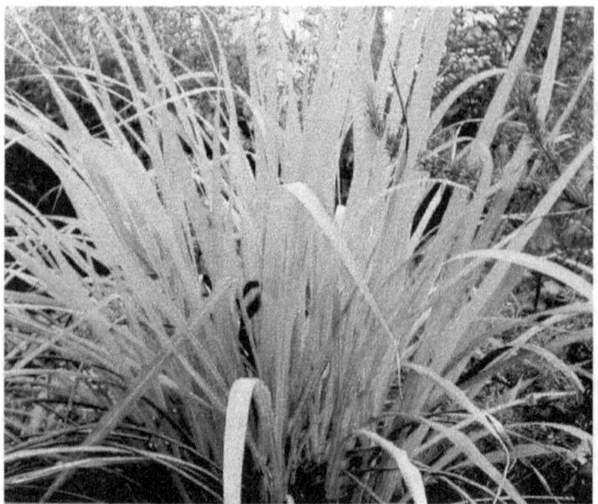

This essential oil allays exhaustion from nerves and stress. It can also help with other conditions from stress.

PATCHOULI (POGOSTEMON CABLIN)

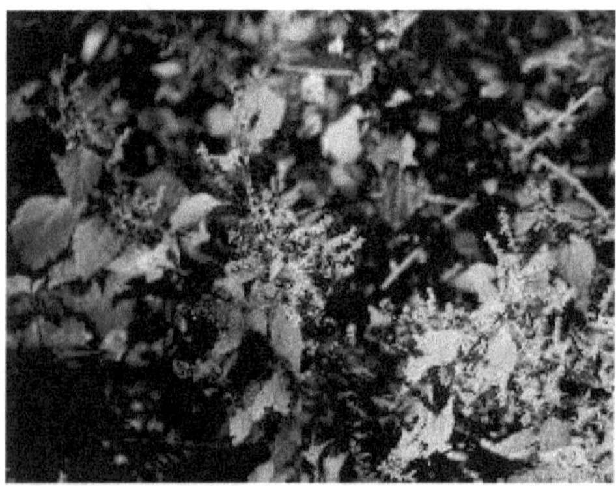

Known for being popular in the sixties, this essential oil helps to calm nerves, and relieve stress.

PETITGRAIN (CITRUS AURANTIUM)

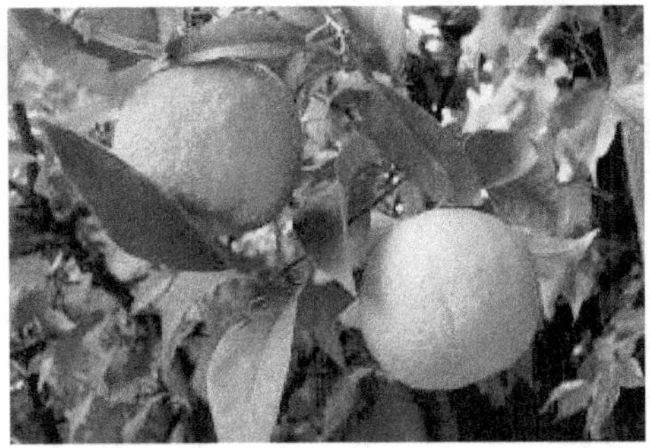

This is another mellow citrus essential oil. It can even out your mood and help with relaxing after a long day.

SANDALWOOD (SANTALUM ALBUM)

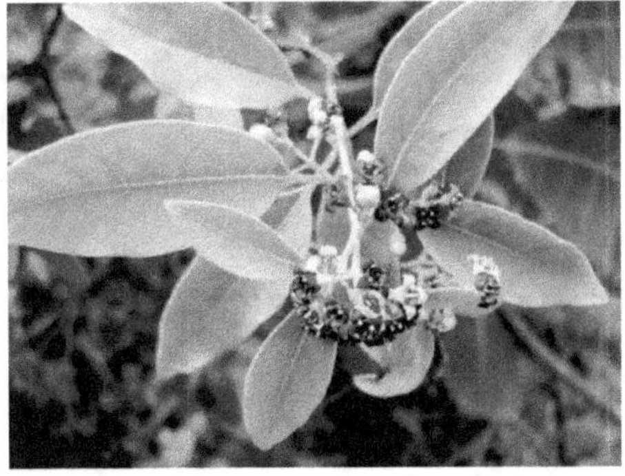

This is one of the most expensive essential oils on the market, second only to Rose, but it is very effective when you're wanting to calm down after a long day, relieve stress from a high stress situation, and it can even help with nervous tension.

After work blend I

.25 oz of Geranium essential oil

.25 oz of Mandarin essential oil

.25 oz of Palmarosa essential oil

After work blend II

.25 oz of Lemon essential oil

.25 oz of Patchouli essential oil

.25 oz of Chamomile essential oil

After work blend III

.25 oz of Sandalwood essential oil

.25 oz of Petitgrain essential oil

.10 oz of Jasmine essential oil

.15 oz of Marjoram essential oil

Chapter 4 - Bath Bombs for Dry Skin

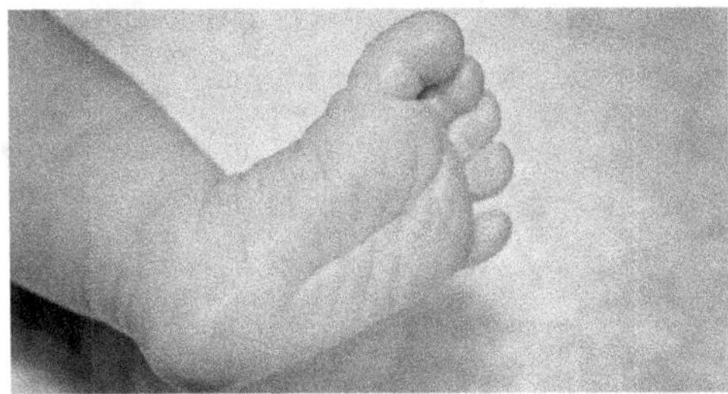

Dry skin can range from being ashen to having psoriasis. Managing your dry skin doesn't have to be a chore. Here are some tips:

1. Don't take scalding hot baths or showers. I know this feels great at the end of the day, but the hot water will dry out your skin, and it only gets worse if you have eczema or psoriasis. Take lukewarm or slightly hot showers and baths instead.

2. Air dry your skin. If you have the time, let the ambient air in your room do the drying for you. It will help moisturize your skin. If you don't have the time, lightly pat your skin dry. Rubbing it dry will irritate sensitive skin.

3. Don't wear tight clothing or clothing with too many dyes. This is especially if you suffer from eczema or psoriasis. There are some dyes that will irritate rashes and plaque patches. Clothing that is too tight will not let your skin breathe and cause irritation as well. Where cotton as much as you can.

4. Sometimes rashes occur as an allergic reaction. The best way to find out about allergies is you schedule an allergy test with your doctor. This will help eliminate any guess work.

5. Keep moisturizer with you at all times. This is important during the winter when the cold air can dry out your skin faster than in the spring or summer.

5. In the case of eczema and psoriasis, find the triggers. Stress can be a big one, but there are many smaller triggers than can be overlooked. Something you ate, changing your detergent, even a new perfume can spark a rash or other skin eruption. Once you learn what caused the episode, you can note it and avoid it in the future.

Essential oils

You will be surprised to find many of the same essential oils here that are used for stress and anxiety. I won't repeat the Latin names, but I will list the most useful ones from above and include how they help with dry skin, eczema and psoriasis.

CHAMOMILE, ROMAN

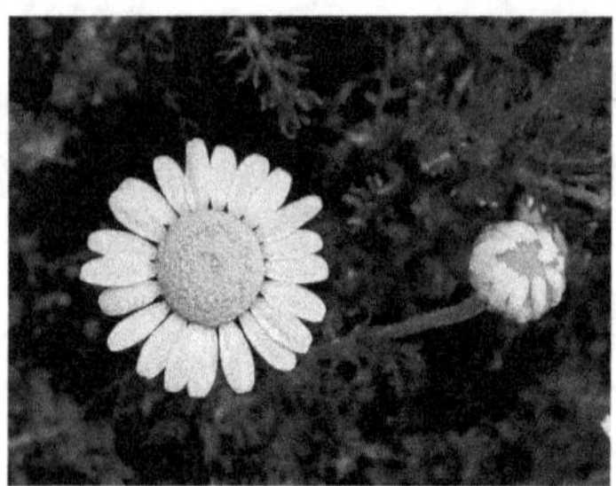

This essential oil helps to reduce inflammation due to skin eruptions, dermatitis, sensitive skin, and eczema.

FRANKINCENSE

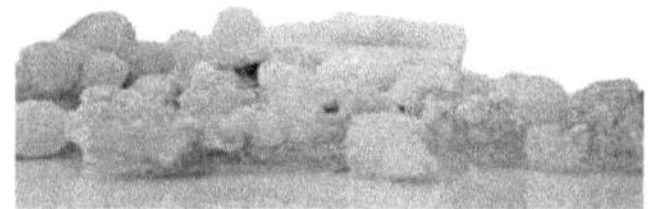

This essential oil can bring a little extra moisture to normally dry skin.

GERANIUM

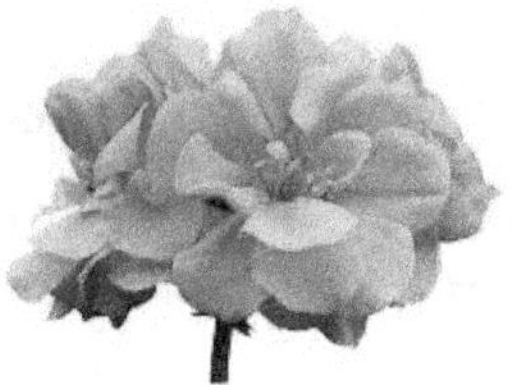

This essential oil is well known for soothing skin irritations, reducing the inflammation due to dermatitis and eczema.

JASMINE

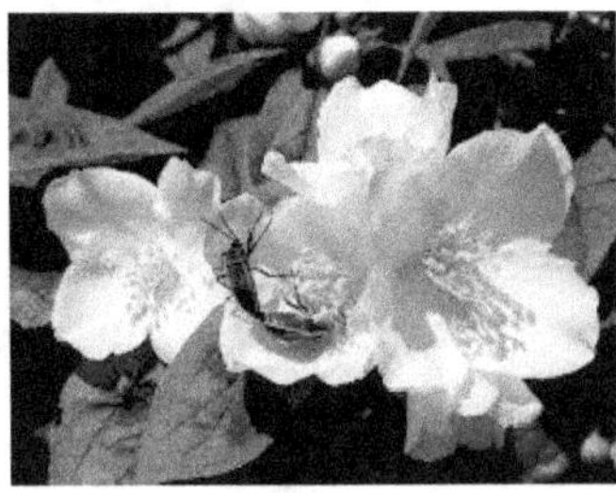

This is a great oil for sensitive or irritated skin.

LAVENDER

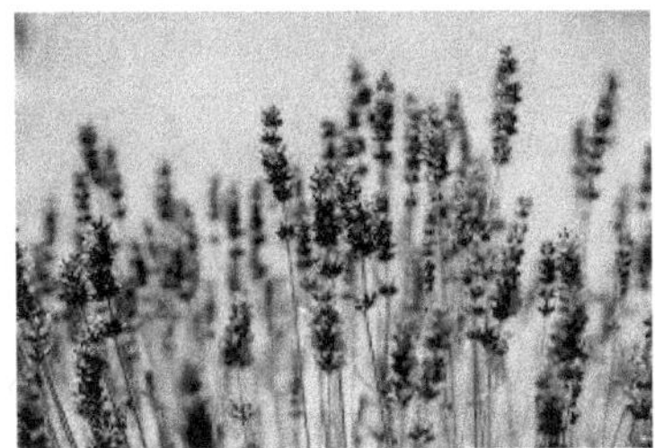

From burns to sensitive skin, to eczema and psoriasis and some many more, this essential oil is great for all skin conditions.

PALMAROSA

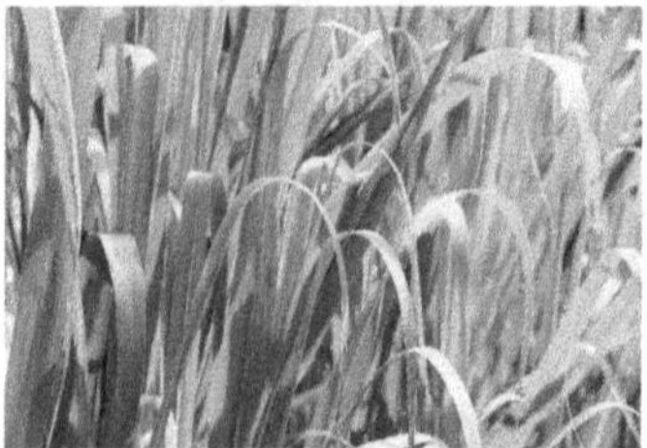

Palmarosa is highly recommended in cases of skin infections as well as dermatitis, eczema, and is well known for moisturizing skin.

PATHCHOULI

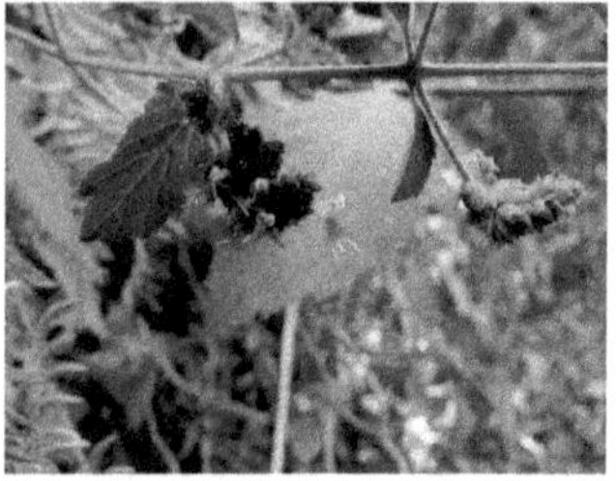

This is the essential oil that is best for weeping eczema and psoriasis. It is also great for treating dermatitis, cracked and chapped skin. It is really good for oily skin.

ROSEWOOD

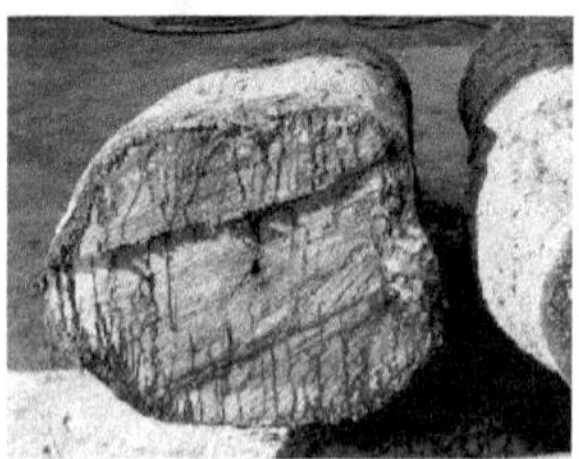

This is another good oil for sensitive skin, dermatitis, and dry skin.

SANDALWOOD

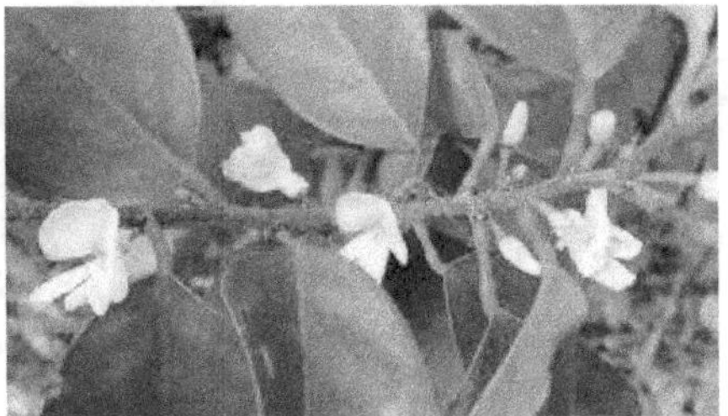

This essential oil is another one that specializes in cracked and chapped skin.

YLANG YLANG

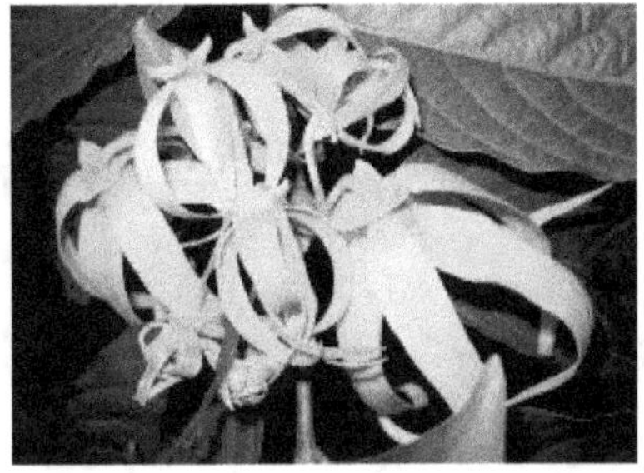

This is often added for blends for general care use. It's also very good for irritated skin, too.

Dry skin I

.25 oz of Lavender essential oil
.25 oz of Ylang Ylang essential oil
.25 oz of Rosewood essential oil

Dry skin II

.50 oz of Palmarosa essential oil
.25 oz of Frankincense essential oil

Dry skin III

.25 oz of Chamomile essential oil
.25 oz of Mandarin essential oil
.25 oz of Jasmine essential oil

Eczema and psoriasis I

.25 oz of Lavender essential oil
.25 oz of Patchouli essential oil
.25 ox of Palmarosa essential oil

Eczema and psoriasis II

.15 oz of Sandalwood essential oil
.10 oz of Patchouli essential oil
.50 oz of Geranium essential oil

Eczema and psoriasis III

.15 oz of Frankincense essential oil
.10 oz of Patchouli essential oil
.25 oz of Chamomile essential oil
.25 oz of Rosewood essential oil

Chapter 5 - Bath Bombs for Oily Skin

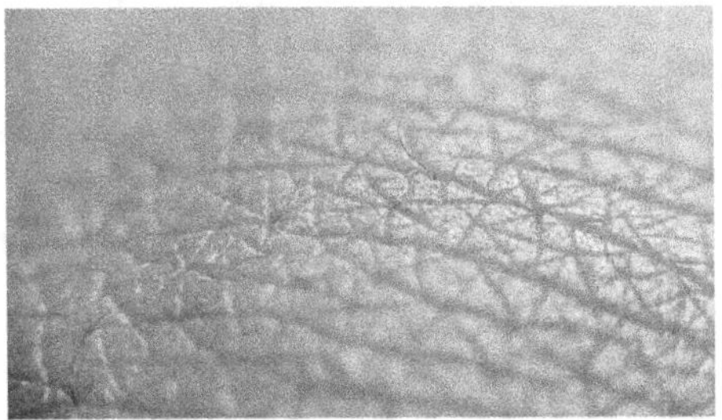

You wash it, turn around a couple of hours later, there it is again, the sheen of the oils showing themselves on your skin. You freshen your makeup, but it comes back. You're at your wit's end on how to handle this, and you're about to throw in the towel, but there are some things you can do to regulate the oils and live a normal life without having to go to extremes.

What if I told you the oily skin you have is due to your body overproducing its own oils in order to keep your skin moisturized? It's true in some cases. Your body produces sebum. This is what keeps you skin soft, supple, and keeps it from drying out. However, in the case of oily skin, your body make more sebum than is needed due to an imbalance. The question would be how to regulate oily skin.

Moisturize after cleansing your face and body. When you're fresh out of the shower or bath, you towel the moisture off of your body. When you apply a moisturizer after to dry off, you are helping your skin stay moisturized, taking the load off the hormones that tell the body to produce it.

There are some essential oils that help with excess sebum production. Top of the list are the citrus based essential oils. So, don't be surprised to see a couple of new names when we get to the recipes, but we have to balance those out with moisturizing essential oils so our body doesn't hit the mass-production button on the sebum.

The citrus essential oils that can help are:

-Bergamot
-Grapefruit: citrus x paradisi This essential oil also helps to tone the skin.
-Lime: citrus aurantifolia
-Mandarin
-Orange blossom/Neroli: (sensitive skin)citrus aurantium
-Petitgrain
-Sweet Orange: citrus sinesis

CEDARWOOD, ATLAS (CEDRUS ATLANTICA)

This oil comes in handy with blemishes and oily skin by reducing the amount of sebum your skin produces. It's a regulator.

CLARY SAGE (SALVIA SCLAREA)

This essential oil helps to regulate the production of sebum as well, but needs to be used in small amounts.

CYPRESS (CUPRESSUS SEMPERVIRENS)

Cypress works to curtail the excess production of sebum. This essential oil is often used in the cases of very oily skin.

FENNEL (FOENICULUM VULGARE)

Fennel helps with oily skin and also helps to bring a healthy glow back to dull skin. This essential oil should be used in small concentrations.

JUNIPER BERRY (JUNIPERUS COMMUNIS)

The oil from this berry helps with oily skin and helps tone the skin as well.

Palmarosa

This one is one another list due to its regenerative properties and because it helps the body regulate sebum production.

Ylang Ylang

Yup, you guessed it. It helps with oily skin, too.

Oily Skin (sensitive)

.25 oz of Sweet orange essential oil
.25 oz of Rosewood essential oil
.25 oz of Cypress essential oil

Oily skin I

.25 oz of Grapefruit essential oil
.25 oz Juniper essential oil
.25 oz of Cedarwood essential oil

Oily skin II

.10 oz of Fennel essential oil
.15 oz of Neroli essenital oil
.25 oz of Palmarosa essential oil

Chapter 6 - Poor Circulation

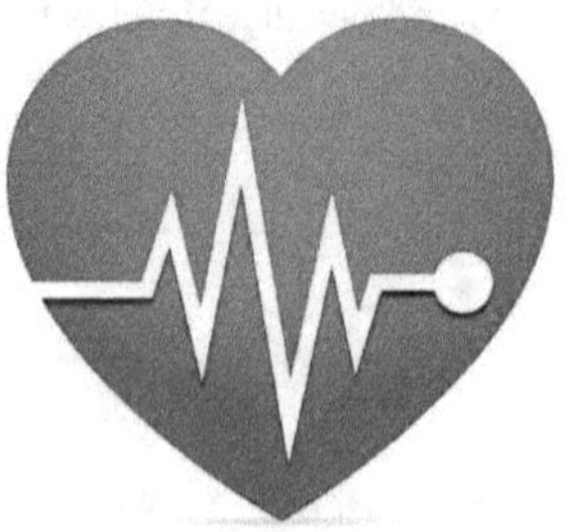

You heart is one of the busiest muscles in your body. It has to make sure enough blood gets pumped through the veins and capillaries so your body can function like it should. As we get older and depending on the jobs we take, it can become a challenge to keep your heart, and the circulatory system as whole, healthy and running the way it should.

Varicose Veins

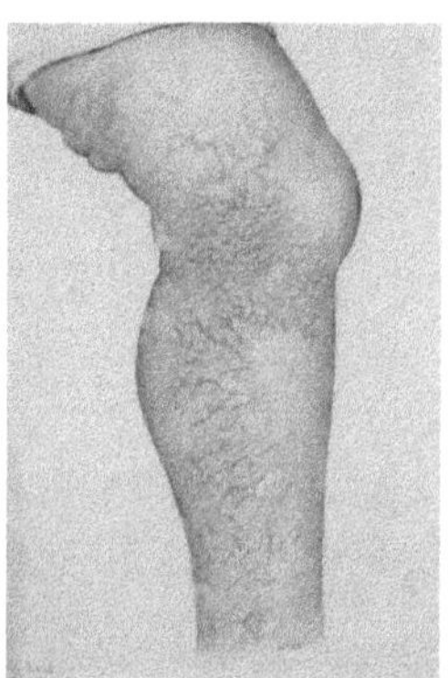

They're purple and bluish and tend to be swollen. I am talking about the veins on your lower legs and feet when you have a job that requires to stand for hours on end. Varicose veins are very common in people who are on their feet most of their working career. This is because being upright add pressure to the veins in those areas, and the more you're walking, standing, or running, the more pressure you put on those veins.

This doesn't happen over time, but over several years. First, the veins become more visible than they used to be. Then, they start looking as if they are going to push through your skin. Finally, the veins look like spider web highways on your legs, forcing you to find ways to cover them up.

Here are some essential oils that are already listed in this book that help with this and other circulatory issues:

Clary Sage, Cypress, Fennel, Geranium, and Lemon.

Here a couple of new ones that help with poor circulation:

LEMON GRASS (CYMBOPOGON CITRATUS)
YARROW (ACHILLEA MILEFOLIUM)

This essential oil also helps to regulate blood pressure and can help in cases of thrombosis and arteriosclerosis.

Varicose veins I

.25 oz of Geranium essential oil
.25 oz of Lemon Grass essential oil
.25 oz of Cypress essential oil

Varicose veins II

.25 oz of Yarrow essential oil
.25 oz of Lemon essential oil
.25 oz of Lemon Grass essential oil

Varicose veins III

.10 oz of Clary Sage essential oil

.15 oz of Fennel essential oil

.25 oz of Lemon Grass essential oil

.25 oz of Yarrow essential oil

Poor circulation

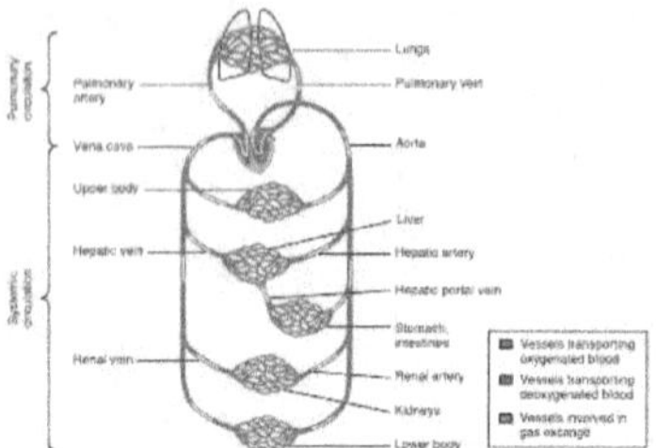

Have your hands and feet gotten cold when you know the room is not chilly? Do have the habit of being chilly when others seem comfortable? You might have poor circulation, and you need to get that checked. Here are some essential oils that work wonders for that. This is, by no means, a definitive list. The number of essential oils that can help with the circulatory system is in the twenties!

CINNAMON (CINNAMOMUM ZEYANICUM)

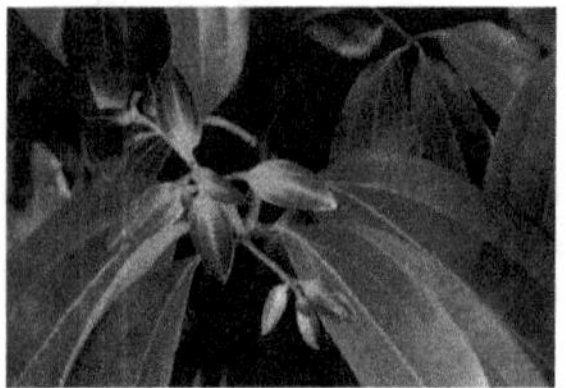

The leaves of this herb are the ones used for the essential oil. It's warming properties help with sluggish and poor circulation as a whole. You can even put three drops to one tablespoon of vegetable oil and rub into your feet in a downward motion to help get the blood flowing.

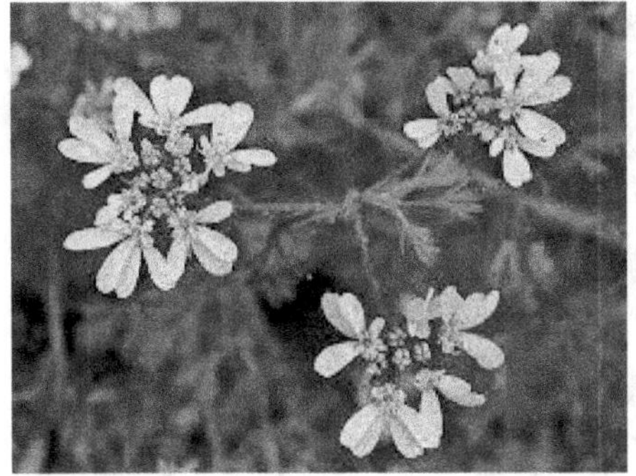

As the Latin name would suggest, it is part of the sage family. It helps with aches and pains as well as poor circulation.

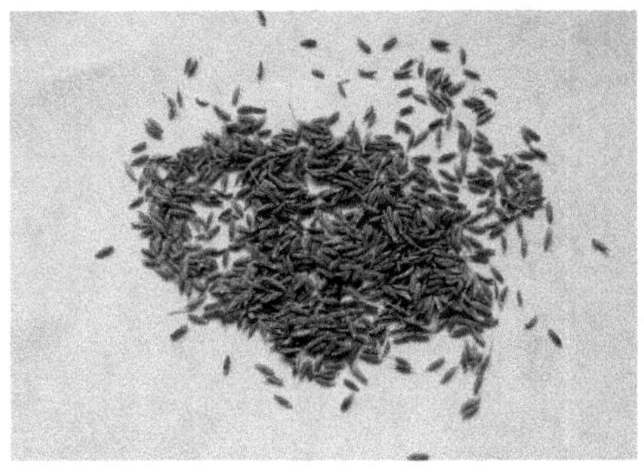

Used widely for cooking in Latin American countries in its herb form, Cumin, as an essential oil, can help with poor circulation.

EUCALYPTUS (EUCALYPTUS GLOBULUS)

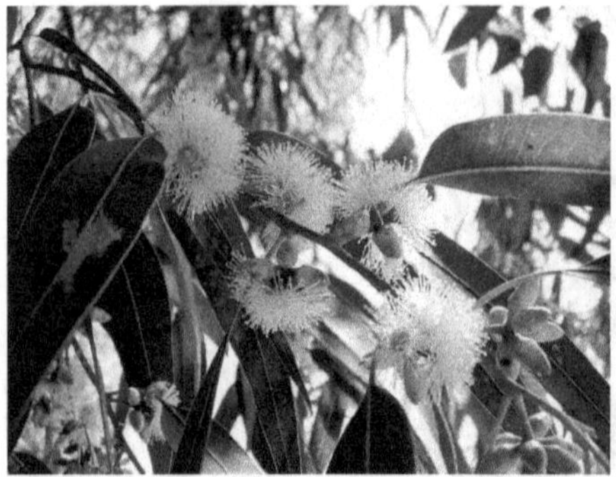

This is another good for poor circulation, but some people tend to be allergic to it.

LIME (CITRUS AURANTIFOLIA)

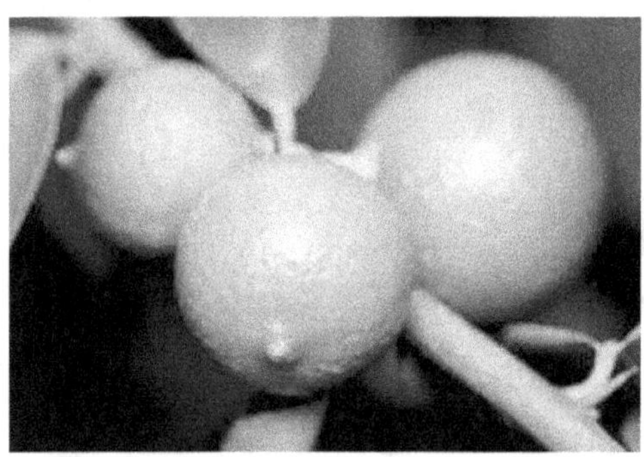

Not only good for skin conditions, but can help with poor circulation and high blood pressure.

ORANGE BLOSSOM (CITRUS AURANTIUM V AMARA)

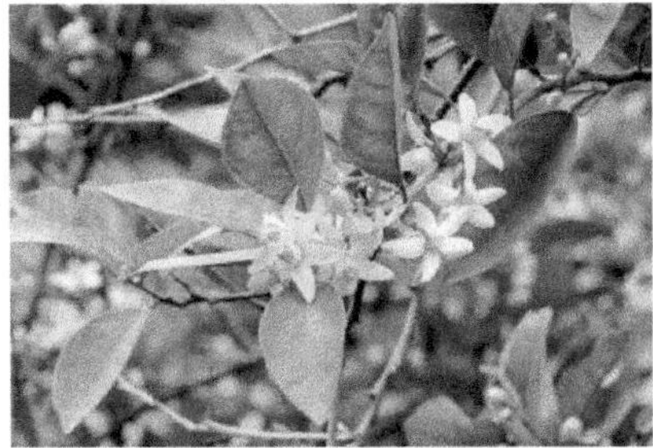

This essential has been used to help with poor circulation and those who has palpitations.

WHITE BIRCH (BETULA ALBA)

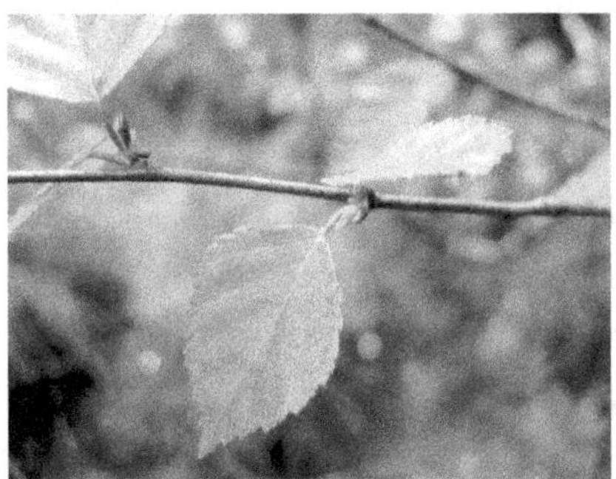

This essential oil is used in blends for poor circulation and edema.

Poor circulation I

.10 oz of Cinnamon Leaf essential oil

.15 oz of White Birch essential oil

.25 oz of Orange Blossom essential oil

.10 oz of Coriander essential oil

.15 oz of Eucalyptus essential oil

Poor circulation II

.25 oz of Orange Blossom essential oil

.10 oz if Cumin essential oil

.15 oz of White Birch essential oil

.25 oz of Lime essential oil

Poor circulation III

.10 oz of Clary Sage essential oil

.15 oz of Fennel essential oil

.25 oz of Orange blossom essential oil

.10 oz of Cumin essential oil

.15 oz of Coriander essential oil

For the heart

For this one, we are going to take a lot of the essential oils from the previous section and chapters. That's right. Most of the essential oils I have already covered are good for heart health. There is only one that I need to elaborate on.

Sweet Orange (citrus senisis)

This one helps with those suffering from heart palpitations.

Heart I

.25 oz of Sweet Orange essential oil

.25 oz of Lavender essential oil

.25 oz of White Birch essential oil

Heart II

.10 oz of Frankincense essential oil

.15 oz of Fennel essential oil

.25 oz of Lemon Grass essential oil

.25 oz of Eucalyptus essential oil

Heart III

.25 oz of Palmarosa essential oil

.10 oz of Cinnamon essential oil

.15 oz of Coriander essential oil

.25 oz of Orange Blossom essential oil

Chapter 7 - Pampering Yourself

Remember when I told you to spoil yourself? This is it. We've gone over a lot of serious issues how you can make bath bombs to help those issues, but now, we're going to have a little fun and learn a few recipes to out and out spoil ourselves.

Mediterranean Breeze

Capture the scent of the Mediterranean with this blend.

.25 oz of Cypress essential oil
.25 oz of Sweet Orange essential oil
.25 oz of Cedarwood essential oil

Tis the Season

.10 oz of Cinnamon essential oil
.15 oz of Fennel essential oil
.25 oz of Frankincense essential oil
.05 oz of Lavender essential oil

Foral Holiday

.25 oz each of Geranium, Ylang Ylang, and Rose.

Conclusion

I hope this book has made it easier for you to start your new hobby and your new way of pampering yourself. There are many more essential oils out there, and I implore you to seek them out and learn about them. You may find a few more to add to your collection and new recipes to try out. Never stop learning!